WHO AM I TO JUDGE?

The Journal of a Pro-Choice Christian Nurse

MsThomasRN

Hov PUBLISHING

Who am I to Judge?
The Journal of a Pro-Choice Christian

HOV Publishing a division of HOV, LLC.
www.hovpub.com
hopeofvision@gmail.com

Cover Design: HOV Design Solutions
Editor: Amy A. Owens for Clarity Communication

Write the Author MsThomasRN at: msthomasrn@gmail.com

For more information about special discounts for bulk purchases, please contact: msthomasrn@gmail.com.

ISBN 978-1-942871-62-0

Library of Congress Control Number:

10   9   8   7   6   5   4   3   2   1

Printed in the United States of America

DEDICATION

I've made many sacrifices along the way, and school was the toughest of them, but it was all worth it. My two small children at the time kept me focused; they were the reason I was devoted to never giving up. Throughout their lives, they have witnessed my struggles and have seen my drive to succeed. Because of them, I am who I am.

My First Born

I dedicate this book to you. I am not sure why God chose me to be your mother, but He did. From the moment I knew about you, I have not had a single regret. You have changed my perception of what life is. You have taught me patience, love, persistence, dedication, and so much more. I love you because you have lit the fire of my desire to be a success and, most importantly, your mom. I pay homage to you, my son, who "they" said would be a high-school dropout, drug dealer, or prisoner. You rejected any negative statistic and showed the world different. You graduated from college and became a productive member of society. Whenever I felt like giving up, your face inspired me to keep on going, and together WE have BEATEN the ODDS!

My Baby Girl

I dedicate this book to you. I never knew how beautiful I was until you came into my life. You have made my life beautiful and bright. You gave me every reason to live life and not give up. I thank God every day for bringing you into my life and blessing me to be your mother.

My Baby Boy

God showed you to me in a dream way before you were thought of. The timing was not perfect then, but He told me you would come. For many years I thought it was just a dream, but then 21 years after your brother, and 18 years after your sister, you presented yourself to me. I became a "born-again mom." You give me so much joy and made my heart melt all over again. Because of you, my journey will continue.

My Family

Mom

You stepped in during the scariest time in my life. Still a baby myself, you made sure I would not fail as a parent. You instilled the value of God, family, education, and work morale into your children. Because of you, my stubbornness to be successful has become my reality. I have the independence and confidence I never thought I would.

Dad

My protector and my foundation. You gave me life. You stepped up to the plate and took on the responsibility of raising me, as well as my children, as your own. You taught me to depend on God and to be responsible for my happiness.

My Sisters

My forever best friends and my crutches. Together, we are a force to be reckoned with. My will to succeed came from watching you both excel.

My Best Friend

You were my comfort during the scariest time in my life. When it seemed no one understood me, you did, and you NEVER passed judgment on me. For this, I love you, and I thank you for always standing in my corner and supporting me.

My Children's Fathers

I thank you for giving me the best gift in the world, my children!

All Medical Providers and Health Care Staff

I thank you for all that you do as supporters of the women's movement. Our jobs are challenging and at times dealing with non-supporters, can make our jobs overwhelming. What I love the most is that regardless of the challenge, we are dedicated to what we do and we stand strong as a community protecting the rights of women. For that, I thank you.

TABLE OF CONTENTS

PREFACE

"I am a "Faith Warrior." My faith in God allows me to step out and rely on Him to direct and redirect my steps. My steps have been ordered, and they have been constant. My obedience has been persistent, and my accomplishments have been great. My continued growth relies on believing that I am covered in His grace and mercy."

MsThomasRN

INTRODUCTION

"The character of a nurse is as important as the knowledge she possesses."

Carolyn Jarvis, MSN, APN, CNP

Throughout my nursing career, I have maintained a keen interest in women's health. My passion for this field comes from my experience as a young mother. I raised two small children on my own while juggling my career, my education, and my family. I've endured some hardships throughout the years, but I was determined to not give up. With faith, dedication to hard work, and persistence, I was able to beat the odds and the negative statistics of being a young black mother. I began my nursing journey as a Certified Nursing Assistant. I worked my way up to the highest level in nursing, becoming the Director of Nursing at a women's health care facility. My stubbornness to achieve my goals gave me the opportunity to experience and witness many things in this nursing field. I vowed to give my children all that I could. For years working hard and making sacrifices became the norm for me, but it was all worth it. My oldest son is a graduate of Hofstra University, pursuing his career in Project Management, while my daughter is a graduate of Brooklyn College and currently pursuing her career in Media and Television Production. I made a promise to myself that the day I made it to the top, I would give back to the very community that afforded me with so many opportunities when I was young. Everyday women, especially those of color, face many obstacles while just trying to live and maintain a "normal life" for themselves and their children. For this reason, I devoted myself to the empowerment of young women facing similar obstacles through any portal I could locate. My career in community public health and women's health has provided me with an excellent experience.

I have worked as a nurse leader, nurse consultant, nurse advocate and nurse educator with various community outreach projects teaching reproductive health and health awareness to young women and men. My enthusiasm and commitment in working with teen women have been even more exciting and rewarding.

The ultimate goal of my career is to provide quality health care services to women and families, of all nationalities. My hope is that empowering these women will have a positive effect on their lives.

I have been asked, "How can you follow the teachings of Christ, call yourself a Christian, and participate in murdering innocent babies?"

Pro-Choice will be defined as "The belief that a woman should have the legal right to abort her unborn child at any point in the pregnancy." Pro-Choice advocates believe abortion is a personal decision and should not be limited by the government or anyone else.

Pro-Life will be defined as "The belief that every human life is sacred and no one, including the mother, has the right to end an innocent life." Pro-Life advocates hold the view that life, from the moment of conception, should be protected.

This book explores my life experience as a pro-choice Christian nurse, my passion and dedication to the women I have chosen to serve. My journey starts from the beginning of my time as a teen mom until this day in time where I continue to serve women. I could have been anywhere in this life given to me by God, but He placed me here. Throughout the trials of my nursing career, I often questioned God as to why He put me in situations that compromised my belief in Him. It took many years to get an answer, and now that I have it, I want to share it with the world. This is my journey as a pro-choice Christian nurse.

CHAPTER 1

This is my Story this is my Song

I was the oldest of three little ladies. My mom "The Backbone of the Family," instilled Christian values within us. Raised in a Christian household, my sisters and I were not strangers to the teachings of Jesus Christ. In fact, we attended church and bible school every Sunday morning, and from Monday through Friday we were learning about God during our school studies. We grew up in a household where the church was not the center of our life, but the Lord was—Momma made sure of that.

At age 7, I started first grade which was the beginning of my Catholic school education. Twelve years of Christian school made the difference in my life; knowing Christ and having a personal relationship with Him as an adult has made me a better person. In a Christian school, religion class was required for every grade, as was attending mass on Wednesdays. Now although I attended Catholic school, I was not Catholic, I was Christian, and I followed the same teachings of Christ just as Catholics, Baptists, and other Christian denominations. It didn't matter one way or the other for us because all students learned the same. However, my sisters and I just did not participate in First Communions and Confessions. When the time came near to complete high school applications, I was told I could go to any high school of my choice as long as it was a Catholic High School, per my mother. My mom was not thrilled with the idea of me attending "public school." I wanted to go to a public high school, one that I knew specialized in nursing. I always knew that I wanted to be a nurse and to attend this school would have afforded me the opportunity to graduate from high school as a Licensed Practical Nurse.

At this time, I felt as if my mom had crushed my dreams. I wanted to become a nurse so badly, that it didn't matter to me where I got my education. I didn't understand at the time, but through my journey, I would soon realize its importance. I chose an all-girls Catholic school to attend and then transferred to another all-girls school. This was a new experience for me because I was used to interacting and learning with males and females. But an all-girls school was not bad. I must say I had so many good times in both high schools I attended. As in elementary school, the rules were the same; religion was a requirement to graduate.

The ladies who attended the school were a cool group, and I quickly developed friendships. I became friends with a young lady and we immediately clicked. We were homeroom buddies, we shared a few classes together, and eventually became best friends in high school. She was special to me because she spoke about Christ and Religion—topics the other ladies didn't speak about. One day while chatting we just began talking about religion and the importance of having Christ in our lives. Who would think that at our age this would be a topic for discussion for us? Now don't get me wrong, we did speak about boys and other things, but religion seemed to be the topic we enjoyed discussing the most. We began reading the Bible and studying it daily. During our lunch break we would spend 3-5 minutes eating and then discussing different chapters from The Bible for the next 40 minutes. After a while, other students started to join in our discussions and soon after we had a lunch room table club of Christian believers. Students would refer to us as 'The Church Gals' but we didn't care because we felt good studying the word.

At this same time, I began to welcome Christ into my life even more. Religion became my favorite thing. Attending my Baptist church every week with my next-door neighbor and good friend became the norm. I also started dating a young man who was the son of a pastor of a Pentecostal church. Our dating days initially consisted of us listening to gospel music and debating the bible. It was different, sex was not a concern as you would think it was with most teenagers. After a year we became more serious with our dating and I became more interested in learning more about the teachings of Christ.

Now you may ask how was it that I was dating a Pentecostal young man, attending a Catholic school, and praising God in a Baptist church. The truth of the matter was that it really didn't matter because all three denominations are one under the Christian faith. We all believe and follow the same teachings of Christ. At age 17, I gave my life to Christ and became a 'Born Again Christian.'

We were dating, but we were strong in our beliefs. I believed in not engaging in any sex activity before marriage and for a long while I stayed true to my beliefs. After dating for a while, things began to get more serious and although we were followers of Christ, we were teenagers; teenagers with raging hormones. We began to engage in activity that was an "abomination" according to The Bible. I hadn't yet had a conversation with my parents as far as sex was concerned; I was inexperienced, naive, and uncertain of the consequences of my actions. We thought that being "careful" without the use of contraception, was okay. For some time, we were lucky but as with anything else, our luck ran out. I missed my menstrual period, and my first pregnancy was at age 17. Afraid of my mother's wrath, we contemplated what we would do. I was in

11th grade at an all-girls Catholic high school and living with my parents. A baby at this time was not an option, but I knew in my heart that getting an abortion was not what I wanted either. I believed that having an abortion would result in some sort of punishment from God. I didn't want to go to hell because I was a murderer. I prayed, I cried, I begged my mother not to make me make a decision I would regret. After a few weeks both our mothers came together and sat us down. They explained to us that raising a child was a physical, emotional, and financial obligation that requires a lot of work and responsibility. We would be held solely accountable for this child. Although my mother did not agree with my decision at that time, she supported my decision under the condition that I complete high school.

My high school allowed me to continue my studies until the end of that school year in June. I must admit it was an uncomfortable experience.

7

Often, I was talked about by the other students and I was constantly stared at. Six months into my pregnancy my stomach was visible and hard to hide. I was told by several teachers, including monks and nuns, to 'cover up,' and that they would 'not glorify' my behavior. Emotionally this pregnancy bothered me while doing my studies because I was the Christian girl who was so in tune with my bible and followings that how dare I do this. I was ashamed for a long while.

Of all my good friends, one friend in particular became my best friend. She was my biggest support during this very scary time in my life. She was my shoulder to cry on and would lift my spirits up when I was down. I later named her as my son's godmother.

My guidance counselor at the time was aware of my situation and was also very supportive. She introduced me to a program that provided free nursing care to young and first-time moms. The program was designed to teach new moms how to be successful parents. I would meet the nurse after school once a week and she would explain to me the importance of a healthy pregnancy and having a healthy baby. It was a great program and very informative.

On September 28, 1991 at 3:47 a.m., I gave birth to my first son. I was an 18-year-old senior in High School. Being a young mom was often a challenge because I did not come first anymore. Everything I did was solely for the benefit of my son.

My mother never gave up on me she was there from the beginning. She made it very clear that although I was the mother of this child, I was still her daughter. I lived in her house and I agreed to follow her rules. Most importantly, I agreed that I would graduate high school and start college. As long as I abided by these rules, she would help me. My mother, this awesome woman, kept her word because I kept mine. Six weeks after I gave birth, I returned to school as a senior. I was even more determined to complete my studies and move forward because I had a child who depended on me. Going back to school and raising a baby was definitely a challenge, even with the help of my family. Some days, I regretted my decision because raising a baby and doing school at the same time was hard work that left little or no time for myself. Most days though, I smiled and pushed myself because the look on my son's face was incentive enough for me to succeed.

I remember one night when my son was 3 months old, at about 11:00 pm he began crying. I was studying for a test the next morning and the crying was continuous and nerve- racking. At the time, I didn't know what was wrong with my son, but I soon discovered that he had colic. Colic occurs when air/gas gets trapped in the infant's intestines. Due to immature abdominal muscles, the infant may not be able to push this air/gas out, this results in abdominal discomfort and a fussing and crying infant for several hours. He cried, for what seemed like an eternity. My mom was in her bedroom next door and did not once come to peak in on me. I did not want to bother my mother because I knew she had to get up early for work. So, I paced up and down in my room, bouncing him and trying to quiet him down. I did this for about a half hour with no relief, until I started to cry because I didn't know what to do. My mother finally came over to my room and peeked in. This was the moment I realized that I was indeed a parent and that this was the REAL deal. She asked me what was going on." I said, "I don't know, he won't stop crying."

She looked at me, looked at him, said, "Okay," and went back into her room. I was puzzled, depressed, and angry all at the same time.

After 2 hours, he finally cried himself to sleep. I was so sleepy and upset that I went to sleep too, ignoring the fact that I had a test in the morning.

The next day, I asked my mom why she didn't come to my rescue. She made it very clear to me, the decision to become a mother was mine not hers. For me to learn how to be a parent, I must figure some things out about motherhood. I had to learn how to interact with my baby, learn his language, his actions, and how to respond to his needs. This is what's known as maternal skills. If you don't respond to your baby, neither you nor your baby wins. She made it very clear that she would always be here if I needed her, but she would not jump in to help me every time. She wanted me to learn how to respond to my infant appropriately in the case that she was not around. From that moment on, my momma made sure that I was developing maternal skills. Whenever my son would cry, she would call my name "Monica, the baby is crying." I quickly learned, and my mother made sure I did not forget that I have a child who demanded my attention at all times… Motherhood.

CHAPTER 2

You are Forgiven my Child

After giving birth to my son, I returned to school to complete my studies. I was now a mom and a student, and I was in a relationship with the father of my child. Juggling all three of these titles at once was often challenging and overwhelming. I started birth control pills six weeks after I gave birth to my son to prevent another pregnancy. It was no secret that we were sexually active and bringing another child into this world was not a good idea at this time. With juggling school, a baby, and a relationship I often forgot to take my birth control pills on time, and I found myself pregnant again.

I was a senior in high school and I had a seven-month-old baby. We were not prepared for another child and, above all, I did not want to disappoint my mother. Against all that my son's father and I believed, we decided to abort this pregnancy. Ashamed of what people would think, I decided to keep this secret. My mother and my son's father were the only two people who knew.

We did some research and found a facility that would perform the procedure for me in a safe and confidential environment. On the day of the procedure, my son's father accompanied me and was there by my side until the very end. I remember feeling so guilty and afraid of the consequences of doing this. Fear made me ambivalent, so I prayed, and I prayed until my heart spoke to my soul saying, "Monica you have come to me with a sincere and pure heart, now let it go, I have already forgiven you." With this answer, I felt a sense of comfort come over me, and I proceeded with my decision to terminate my pregnancy.

15

1 John 1:8-9 (KJV) tells us, *"If we confess our sins, he is faithful and just to forgive us our sins, and to cleanse us from all unrighteousness."*

CHAPTER 3

"A" Day

On the day of my procedure, my partner and I arrived at the facility and after counseling, it was my time. I was afraid, anxious, and overwhelmed all and I could feel my heart pounding through my chest. I remember the nurse who brought me into the room, she was a pleasant older nurse and she was nice to me. I told her I was scared and she addressed my fears about the procedure and did the one thing I NEVER expected her to do. She wrapped her arms around me and began to pray over me. "Father God take this young lady into your arms and protect her. Lord, you said that if man come to you and ask for forgiveness with a genuine heart that you would forgive them. Let thy will be done, we ask all these things in your name, Amen."

Tears fell from my eyes, and she took a napkin and began to wipe my face. She said "My child I am here with you. I will not let you walk alone; you will overcome this. I will be here when you finish." At that very moment, just minutes before I walked into the operating room, I felt a sense of calm and peace. She walked me to the operating room and continued to hold my hand until I fell asleep. After the procedure was complete, I rested in the recovery room for a while. When I woke up, she was there by my side as she promised.

This lady had such an impact on me. I wouldn't have thought that years later I would follow in her footsteps. Why would God put a religious, Christian nurse in this field? Was she an angel? I don't know. As baffled and confused as I was, I will be forever grateful that she was present at that time. She helped me get through a traumatizing experience by convincing me that God had already forgiven my transgressions. Before I left the facility, she pulled me to the side again and told me something I'd never forget. She said, "My child you are special and you are beautiful. You are destined to be great one day. Today you have a clean slate, your sins have been removed, and you are free to carry on. What happened today was already written in your life book to take place. God knows all things and approves all things. You were given a second chance. Go in peace and leave your burdens and worries at this door when you leave this facility. I don't know you, but I know you worship a mighty God. Let His will be done. I will see you in two weeks for your check up." That nurse's name was Nurse Sara.

In two weeks, I returned for my follow-up as recommended and the first person I asked for was Nurse Sara. The receptionists at the front desk said that she was not there that day. Again, confusion covered my face, because she told me that she would see me two weeks and I was hoping to see her. While seeing the medical provider for my follow-up I asked when Nurse Sara would be back. The provider told me that Nurse Sara suffered a stroke and would not be back to work. I asked if there was any way I could contact her to thank her and I was told that she passed. I stood there speechless, confused, and lost all at the same time. I could not believe this. She was just here and now she was gone. I never got the chance to tell her thank you for being there for me during this difficult time. All I could do is just remember her goodness and the way she supported me through a very difficult moment in my life. As I spoke with the provider, I heard his voice, but I retained nothing, and nothing registered, because all I kept thinking about was Nurse Sara.

It took me time to recover and reflect on what I had just done. I did what Nurse Sara told me to do and tried to put this behind me, but it was very difficult, and I had a hard time dealing with it. After a few weeks and prayer, I was able to pull myself together. I still had a baby boy to care for and school to attend. Other than my mom and son's father, I eventually told my best friend about my pregnancy and abortion experience. As with all things, she was understanding and most importantly non-judgmental. She was my sister in Christ and was there for me without question, and that's why, I will always appreciate and love her beyond words.

CHAPTER 4

My Calling

Two months after this experience I graduated high school in the fall, I started college to pursue my career in Nursing. I always knew I wanted to be a nurse; I just never knew what field I wanted to practice in. I admired the women in my life that helped me during pregnancy and beyond, so I decided that I wanted to help women who were in the same situation I was in. I wanted to be a role model for women, educating and mentoring them on wellness, life, and their reproductive health.

The genuine and sincere response these ladies—my mother, my guidance counselor, my best friend and Nurse Sara—gave me I wanted to reciprocate to other women. So, I decided to dedicate and devote my Nursing Career to practicing in Women's Health.

Nursing was a challenge. College was a challenge. Now I had two small children. The combination of all three was an enormous challenge. I had some struggles during my nursing studies, but I was determined to not give up. With the support from my family, I graduated and became the nurse I always wanted to be.

In my first nursing job, I worked as a staff nurse at a nursing home and rehabilitation facility. I worked there for a few years while acquiring medical and surgical training with the geriatric community. The pace of learning was appropriate, appreciated, and prepared me for the more complicated nursing that I wanted to do. I loved the operating room and I loved women's health, my dream was to combine the two and work as a nurse in gynecological surgery. I had an organization in

23

mind that I wanted to work for, but I did not have the qualifications I needed to work there. So, with the help of my supervisor at the nursing home, I went back to school to continue my nursing journey. She provided me with two nursing scholarships to help with my studies which came in handy and helped me as I was providing for two small children. I went back to school to become a registered nurse. This was the nursing qualification that I needed to apply for the job I wanted.

After graduating again, I applied for a job as a surgical nurse at a worldwide known facility that provides women's health care. Initially, I did not get the job, but I was so determined to be a part of this organization that I applied several more times and followed up every week, until they decided to hire me.

Finally, I was doing what I enjoyed most which was educating and providing health care to women. From this point on I was determined to live out my dream as a women's health care provider and excel to the highest level as a Director of Nursing overseeing gynecological surgical services. After two decades of experience, dedication, and persistence, I made my dream a reality and became the Director of Nursing of Gynecological Surgical Services despite all the odds against me. This title gave me the permission to groom my nursing staff as professional, humble, sincere, compassionate, and non-judgmental nurses. There are not many nursing professionals who choose to work in this field but the ones who do, choose to because of the qualities they possess for servicing women.

CHAPTER 5

A Pro-Choice Nurse

Being a pro-choice Nurse means that I support a woman's right to choose what she desires to do with her body. She has the legal right to terminate an undesired pregnancy and the right to access reproductive health care without being punished for her personal choices. For over 20 years I have been an advocate for women regardless their race, religion and/or status in life. I have been asked, "How can you follow the teachings of Christ, call yourself a Christian and participate in murdering innocent babies?" My response has always been consistent.

"Being pro-choice is my choice and caring for women is what I've been called to do. I do my job with a sincere heart, a non-judgmental spirit, and the courage to positively impact the lives of the women I service. I will continue to do what I've been called to do because I love what I do!"
Ms. Thomas, RN

I found my place in nursing. I fell in love with women's health and I have made myself available to service women through any portal I could. My journey in this field has been the best experience ever. Working with women of all ages and cultures has been a truly amazing and rewarding experience for me. To be able to empower and change the lives of women for the past 20 years is what I dedicate myself to every day when I put on my nursing uniform. This book is a testimony to women who may not understand why God places them in certain situations. Be assured that it is for a reason. Your story has already been written. Learn not to question God but learn that in order for you to excel in life, there's a journey and process that must take place first. To tell your story, you must travel through your journey first.

The faces of the thousands of women who have crossed my path remain with me. I forget their names, but their stories will forever be in my thoughts and in my heart. The community of abortion-care nurses is extremely small. Not many nurses care to participate in this field for personal reasons. Initially, I was afraid of what I would see or how I would feel as a contributor to this care, but with time and prayer I've learned to separate my emotions so that I can provide passionate care to my patients.

The topic of abortion has always been a sensitive one. The nursing professionals in this field are represented by a small percentage of women and men who choose this career. We work with the understanding that health and reproductive rights are essential to women's health and well-being. Although there are many arguments and debates behind abortion care, we provide our patients with the information and support they need to have this procedure done in a safe, comfortable, and confidential environment. It is our moral responsibility to protect our patients and respect their choices.

Providing safe abortion care prevents unsafe abortions and deaths. In many countries, abortion practice is illegal. However, it is possible to find a provider who will perform an abortion for cheap, but in an unsafe manner that may cost a woman her life. Women often suffer at the hands of these providers resulting in serious harm, infection, or even death. I am glad that although abortion care is a sensitive topic, I live in a country where it can be performed in a safe environment. My colleagues are of different nationalities and religions but in this field, we come together as one because we believe in one mission only, and that is to support women's rights.

CHAPTER 6

Women's Reproductive Health Rights

A woman's reproductive rights gives her the legal right to make decisions for herself regarding her reproductive health and the care she receives, including the right to safe, legal, and judgment-free abortion, contraception, and sexual education.

According to the World Health Organization, "[Reproductive] rights rest on the recognition of the basic rights of all couples and individuals to decide freely and responsibility the number, spacing and timing of their children and to have the information and the means to do so, and the right to attain the highest standard of sexual and reproductive health. They also include the right of all to make decisions concerning reproduction free of discrimination, coercion and violence."

The choice to abort a pregnancy is NEVER easy but having the right to choose is what gets her through. Just imagine if your rights as a woman were taken away and you were forced to carry an undesired pregnancy. In the United States during the1960s (the women's movement) women fought for their reproductive rights.

Norma McCorvey, also known as Jane Roe, terminated an unwanted pregnancy in the late 1960s in Texas. At this time abortions were only legal when done to save the life of the woman. For a termination done for a reason other than that, a woman resorted to finding a medical provider who would perform this practice illegally for a fee in an undisclosed, secret location. Women tolerated the excruciating pain of the procedure, and then were often left to fend for themselves afterwards; even if that meant they hemorrhaged or suffered from a post-abortion infection.

According to the Guttmacher Institute, in the 1950s and 1960s, the estimated number of illegal abortions in the U.S. ranged from 200,000 to 1.2 million per year. This marked the movement of legalizing abortions and changing the law. In 1970, the attorneys filed a lawsuit on the behalf of McCorvey and all the other women "who were or might become pregnant and want to consider all options," against Henry Wade, who was against abortions. This legal case became known as Roe vs. Wade. Abortion had already been legalized in Hawaii and New York State since 1970, and soon after in Alaska and Washington. The tide was turning for women's reproductive rights.

In January 1973, the Supreme Court granted the motion to overturn the abortion law across the nation because it violated constitutional right to privacy. The court declared that abortion was implicit in the right to privacy protected by the 14th Amendment. Legalizing abortion federally now meant that women had the right to terminate undesired pregnancies. Fast forward to today, abortion practice has advanced with the help of technology. Women can choose from several types of abortion procedures. Regardless the procedure chosen, women are safe, cared for by passionate health staff, and counseled and educated regarding preventive care.

CHAPTER 7

Abortion

Every year in the United States, women of all ages, races, nationalities, and religions terminate a pregnancy for reasons unknown. According to the Centers for Disease Control, "A legal induced abortion is defined as an intervention performed by a licensed clinician (e.g., a physician, nurse-midwife, nurse practitioner, or physician assistant) that is intended to terminate an ongoing pregnancy."[1]

The decision to terminate a pregnancy is difficult and highly personal but it does not have to be a traumatic experience. Technology and medical

---

[1] https://www.cdc.gov/reproductivehealth/data_stats/abortion.htm

research have found ways to perform this procedure safely and effectively by way of several options.

A.   Medical Abortion

A medical abortion is a non-surgical medical procedure performed in a doctor's office, clinic or hospital intended to end an early pregnancy. This procedure is performed under the discretion of a board certified and licensed medical provider. Before this procedure is performed, a complete medical history of the patient is taken, a sonogram is done to confirm the pregnancy, a psychological evaluation is conducted, and the patient's consent is obtained.

A medical abortion allows the woman to terminate her pregnancy in private. Some women choose this abortion for fear of pain and the experience of having a surgical procedure. A medical procedure is less invasive and gives the woman more control over her body going through this process.

1. The first medication given to the patient is Oral mifepristone (Mifeprex). This medication is provided by a medical provider and taken at the providers office. According to Mayo Clinic (2018), "Mifepristone (mif-uh-PRIS-tone) blocks the hormone progesterone, causing the lining of the uterus to thin and preventing the embryo from staying implanted and growing. This medication takes a few hours to work and can cause some mild side effects like abdominal discomfort and vaginal bleeding. Patients are encouraged to be in safe place a few hours after taking this medication. The patient is instructed to take the second medications within hours, or days later.

2. Misoprostol (my-so-PROS-tol) or Cytotec is the second medication given to this patient. She is instructed to self-administer this medication at

home, hours or days after taking mifepristone. This medication is slowly dissolved buccally (cheek) or inserted into the vagina. This medication causes the uterus to contract and bleed expelling the embryo (no visible body parts) through the vagina. This process can cause intense cramping and bleeding. The patient is advised to remain in a safe place and to take pain medication for relief.

The Food and Drug Administration (FDA) has approved the use of these medications up to 10 weeks of pregnancy. A follow-up exam approximately a week later is scheduled before the patient leaves this appointment; it ensures the abortion procedure was completed and addresses any concerns the patient may have.

B. Surgical Procedure

A surgical abortion is an invasive procedure that uses a suction method to terminate a pregnancy and empty the uterus. This procedure, from beginning to end, can take 10-30 minutes depending on the stage of the pregnancy. The patient can elect to use: (1) local anesthesia where they remain awake and are given local pain medication via the cervix for relief; (2) moderate sedation where they remain awake and are given intravenous (IV) pain and relaxing medications for comfort prior to the procedure; or (3) general anesthesia where they are given IV medication and are put to sleep while the procedure is performed. Whichever procedure is chosen, the patient will have minimal bleeding and may feel cramping during or after the procedure. Pain management options are available and discussed prior to the procedure. Providing there are no complications, after the procedure recovery is quick. At the discretion of the registered nurses, the patient will need to wait in the clinic until they have been assessed and it is determined it is safe for her to leave (approximately 30-60 minutes). Prior to discharge, the patient is given discharge instructions and advised of side effects to expect afterwards.

Regardless of the woman's choice, the decision to terminate a pregnancy is highly personal and can be extremely difficult. For this reason, no matter what procedure is chosen, every woman is counseled after the procedure. It is our responsibility as nurses to provide discharge-care instructions, words of comfort, and assurance to patients as they transition through this stage.

CHAPTER 8

Saturday Mornings

Saturday mornings were always interesting when I walked into my job. Just about every Saturday there were abortion activists who stood in front of the building targeting young women (preferably those women of color). They were a small group of elderly women who carried their bibles, their rosaries, and pamphlets on why women should not terminate their pregnancies. They displayed horrific pictures of unborn babies and sometimes they were bold enough to scream at patients as they entered the building. Occasionally, they offered prayer with the young women, but their main goal was to prevent women from terminating their pregnancies. Showing horrific pictures of unborn fetuses was a scare tactic they often used.

From my experience, they were not very successful. Patients still came in and often shared their experience with me on how uncomfortable they felt as they walked into the building because of the persistent and arrogant abortion activists outside. Often, these patients would take the pamphlets given to them and continue walking into the building. These women had their minds made up way before they came to the facility. As hard as the decision was for them, they had a reason and a right to their choice.

One Saturday, I stopped and spoke to one of these ladies, because I wanted to know exactly what they told the patients who would stop and listen to them. The old lady asked me if I was going in that building to kill my baby. She told me that if I terminated my pregnancy, by killing an innocent child my soul would dwell in the pit of fire after my life here on earth. She told me that I would be labeled as a 'killer' in God's book and that God would never forgive me. There would be no way possible for me to redeem my soul.

She told me that if I choose to continue my pregnancy that she would refer me to programs that could assist me with my pregnancy and help financially when my baby was born. She told me that God would provide for me and my child. I did not speak, I just listened as this lady spoke to me. She gave me multiple pamphlets some with prayer scriptures on it and others with the horrific pictures of unborn babies. She told me to think about the choice I was about to make because it would determine my presence in my after-life. I took the information she gave along with a plastic rosary she gave me, and I proceeded into the building. She watched me in disgust as I walked into the building. If looks could kill, I'd be dead.

I was never mad at the activist for their beliefs, because everyone is entitled to their opinion. The problem I had was that most times they used and twisted "selected verses" from the Bible to make patients feel bad not considering patient's choice to terminate their pregnancy. They acted as if they were innocent and without sin. The Bible says:

"Let he that is without sin cast the first stone."
John 8:7

The next Saturday, I stopped again to speak with the same little old lady. I had to remind her who I was and that we spoke last Saturday. After a few moments of thinking, she remembered who I was. She smiled initially and then she frowned because she remembered me walking into 'that building.' She asked me if I changed my mind about terminating my pregnancy. Now, remember I was a nursing employee at this facility and I was not pregnant. I wanted to know what patients were being told, so this time I did most of the speaking. I kindly explained to her that I was not pregnant and that I was a "Pro-Choice Christian" I told her that I did not appreciate her wrongfully quoting the bible for her benefit. I asked her if she was without sin…but she had no answer. I asked her if she was a member of the Supreme Court, she told me no, so I asked her "Then who are you to judge me and the choices that I make?" According to the bible you carry every Saturday morning, it says:

"Judge not, and ye shall not be judged: condemn not, and ye shall not be condemned: forgive, and ye shall be forgiven." Luke 6:37

"Be it known unto you therefore, men and brethren, that through this man is preached unto you the forgiveness of sins: And by him all that believe are justified from all things, from which ye could not be justified by the law of Moses." Acts 13:38-39

BOOK 2

Testimonies

Lord, I ask that as I start my day, you give me compassion, understanding, and strength as I service the many women who cross my path today. I ask that you place power in my hands to heal, and that you place comfort in my voice to soothe the pain. Enable me to give those who are lost hope and those who are weak strength to get through this day.

I ask all these things in your name,

Amen.

CHAPTER 9

Her Womb, Her Choice

"Women are not an interest group. They are mothers, and daughters, and sisters, and wives, they are half of this country and they are perfectly capable of making their own choices about their health." President Barack Obama

This book is dedicated to the thousands of women who have crossed my path throughout my journey as a Reproductive Health Nurse. I've chosen to share with you the testimonies of several of those women and the reasons why they decided to terminate their pregnancies. The decision to end a pregnancy is never an easy one. For some women it is the hardest decision they'll ever make in their life, especially if the pregnancy was planned. For some women, it may be a decision made to save their own lives, and for others it may be a decision of convenience. Either way, these decisions mentally, emotionally, financially, and/or physically take a toll on the women who is undergoing this procedure. In New York State there is a process that takes place when a woman decides to terminate her pregnancy. A woman is supported from the moment she decides to terminate until she completes the process, and beyond. There are many states that do not support women and their reproductive rights like New York. I've witnessed many women from other states and other countries who have come here to have this procedure performed because of the support they know they will receive coming here. The next chapter of this book will give you a better understanding of why reproductive rights to women are imperative to her well-being. A man will NEVER understand the emotional process a woman goes through when an abortion is performed. Throughout my journey, I have crossed paths with several women that have touched my soul. Looking back, I thank God that he gave me the necessary tools and skills I needed to be a blessing to these women during their time of need. After learning why God appointed me to do this task, I accepted my calling and made a promise to God and myself that I would continue my purpose as a reproductive nurse. Here are the testimonies of several woman I have serviced along my journey.

CHAPTER 10

A Product of Rape

"RAPE is never DESERVED, it is never ASKED FOR, it's never the fault of THE SURVIVOR."

(Author Unknown)

Imagine being forced to carry a pregnancy that was conceived by rape. No woman should ever have to go through that trauma. According to Connecticut Alliance to End Sexual Violence, "Each year, an estimated 25,000 American women will become pregnant following an act of sexual violence. As many as 22,000 of those pregnancies could be prevented through the prompt use of emergency contraception."[2]

---

[2] https://endsexualviolencect.org/resources/get-the-facts/national-stats/

I have worked with many professional women in this field. When I expressed a desire to write this book, one of my colleagues came to me and asked me to include her testimony. Until then her story had never been told to any of her colleagues, I was the first. She said sharing her story helps her to continue her healing process although it has been many years since she was given this information. She shared her story and her reasons for becoming a nurse in a field that constantly reminds her of her struggles to cope.

My colleague was the product of a sexual attack. At the very young age of 13, my colleague's mother was raped by a family friend. According to my colleague, her mother did not report the rape at that time because she was threatened by her attacker. Who would have believed her story? She kept this secret to herself never realizing that she was pregnant. As time went by my colleague's grandmother noticed a change in her daughter's

51

body. When her grandmother took her daughter to the doctor, they were presented with the news that my colleague's mother was six months pregnant. The first thought was to abort the pregnancy, but she was too far along and, in a state, where abortion services were hard to find. She had no choice but to continue her pregnancy.

After hours of questioning, her daughter finally broke her silence and shared her story with authorities. Her mother learned that not only was her daughter raped and threatened but was also forced to carry this pregnancy to term. The family member responsible for this was eventually arrested and jailed for sex with a minor as well as additional charges.

My colleagues' mother was just 13 years older than her. Her mother knew nothing about taking care of a baby, so she decided to give her child up for adoption to a woman who had difficulty conceiving a child. When my colleague was 20 years old, her adoptive family told her the truth about her life. My colleague said although she was very grateful to her adopted family for loving and raising her as their own, she felt lost, empty, and for years lived with regret. She never married and never had children. She decided to search for her biological mother because there were questions that only she could answer. After two years of searching, she found her mother. My colleague's biological mother told her that she was raped by a family friend and that she hid her pregnancy from her mother because the rapist threatened her life. She told my colleague when she found out how far along the pregnancy was, it was too late to abort the pregnancy. She said, there were not many places that would do safe abortions for young women in that state back then. She had heard so many horrible stories of women dying after having unsafe abortions that she was afraid, so she was forced to continue her pregnancy. She knew that she could never love her the way she wanted because of the way she was conceived, so she decided to give her away to a family who would love her unconditionally. "I was 13 years old, I knew nothing about raising a baby, I was too young to work, and I only had a sixth-grade education, I could not keep you because in my heart I knew I would not love the way you deserved, but I loved you enough to let you go." Harsh words to swallow but my colleague told me she respected her mother for being honest and telling her the truth. My colleague says she is appreciative to her birth mother for continuing her pregnancy and giving her to a loving family. Since then my colleague decided to continue her relationship with her biological mother.

After hearing her story, I questioned my colleague as to why she decided to work in an environment that reminded her daily what she was, a product of rape. She expressed to me that she

54

wanted to be an advocate for women with similar stories and to protect the reproductive rights of those women. After learning her history, she decided to return to nursing school, become a Registered Nurse and work in the women's health field. She said she made a promise to herself that she would no longer live her life in regret, instead she'd be a voice and an advocate for women who were victims of rape. She has been an abortion nurse for the past 30 years and she says, "Working as an abortion nurse allows me to provide sensitive care to women in these situations. Having an abortion does not make you a bad person, giving your child up for adoption doesn't make you a bad person, no woman should have to live their life in regret, doubt or fear. I choose to turn this negative energy into a positive force and that's why I'm so passionate about being here providing care for these women."

"Healing is not an overnight process. It is a daily cleansing of pain; it is daily healing of your life."

Leon Brown

CHAPTER 11

Single Mom

One story I will never forget was my very first counseling session 19 years ago. A 24-year-old single mother of four children who was 12 weeks pregnant with her fifth child came to the clinic and I happened to be her nurse. After she was financially processed, a sonogram was performed, and she was next in line to be counseled by me. Normally a counseling session would take 15-20 minutes, but her session lasted 40 minutes. Her story touched my soul so much that it was one I would always remember. As I mentioned, she was a single mom of 4 children and her sonogram report revealed that she was 12 weeks pregnant with twins. When I told her, she had a twin gestation she broke down in tears. "OMG, I can't believe this! God why would you do this to me?" This lady cried hysterically questioning God for what seemed an eternity in my office. I leaned over to this lady, embraced her in my arms and together we cried and began to talk to God. After sobbing for 15 minutes, she asked me to give her a minute to think about what she wanted to do, so I stepped out. When I came back in the room, she had dried her tears and refocused. With a stern face she looked at me and said, "I'm ready to proceed." I asked her if she was positively sure in her decision, she said "Yes," and then proceeded to tell me her story: "Nurse Monica, I have 4 small children—ages 1, 3, 5 and 9—that I can barely take care of. I have no family here that will help me care for my children, so I live in a shelter. Three years ago, I was diagnosed with a lethal disease, I am HIV positive. My last two children have been covered in God's grace and are HIV negative. I didn't live a good life."

At 14-years-old, I ran away from home because I did not get along with my mother. Before I ran away, my mother would bring random men into our home and sleep with them while my brother and I were in the next bedroom. One day, one of those men came to our house while my mother was at work and asked if he could wait for my mother to come home. He had been to the house several times, he was well mannered, yet seductive. I was in the living room at the time, laying across my couch and watching television. He picked my legs up, sat down and put my legs on top of his lap. I thought nothing of this until he began caressing my legs. I felt uncomfortable, but I didn't ask him to stop because it felt good and I was mad at my mother at this time. While he continued stroking my legs, he began talking to me about his job. He asked me if I worked and if not, did I want a job. He told me that I didn't need any experience, I just had to dance and be able to entertain men. He told me the money was fast, easy and plentiful. He told me that

I can start whenever I wanted. I agreed, and to seal our agreement he gave me a $50 bill, just like that.

The next day he invited me to a strip club where he worked and that's when it all went downhill. The first night I was nervous, but I soon warmed up after realizing how easy the money came. The first gentleman I encountered asked for a five-minute lap dance. After I was done the gentleman handed me a $100 bill and said thank you. That night I made $600 in four hours. I became addicted to the fast and easy money. Sex and money became my life. I was living the good life and loving every minute of it. My mother's friend made me promise not to tell my mother what was going on and I agreed. Every day I went to the strip club and everyday was a good pay day. I was still living at home and my mother's friend was still coming over as if nothing was going on. After a few weeks, I got more and more comfortable and my mother's friend approached me with a new proposal. He told me I needed a pimp, someone to watch my back while I was working. He told me that he could take care of me, manage my money and my clientele. Again, I agreed and the next thing I knew I was working for this man and giving him a portion of my money every night. I was ok with that because he was good to me. My mother found out what was going on and we got into a physical fight. I left the apartment, never to return. As promised, he took care of me and allowed me to stay with him at his apartment. We eventually became intimate and soon after we became a couple. He was much older than I, but I didn't care, he was good to me. I lived with this man for four years and when I turned 18 years old, he married me.

I got pregnant soon after we got married and then again with my second child, a few years after that. When I got pregnant for the third time, I also found out that I contracted HIV. My husband was not an honest man, but I knew this. I was devastated, but I decided to keep my pregnancy and by the grace of God my third child was born HIV negative. My last child was a surprise, but again I decided to keep this pregnancy. I gave birth to my daughter who was also born HIV negative. With all the children I now had, and my bad health, I couldn't work as much. Some days depending on how I felt I couldn't get out of bed. My husband eventually grew sicker and sicker and then one day his heart gave out. Here I was HIV positive, four children to care for, no job, in and out of the hospital, living in a shelter, and no family support. I hit rock bottom. After my husband passed, I found out I was pregnant again, so here I am."

After telling me her life story she broke down crying again. She said, "As much as I want to keep these babies, having them will either kill me or compromise my health in a way that I cannot take care of my other children. I take 10-15 pills of medication a day. I have my good days and I have my bad days. On my bad days, I depend on my 9-year-old daughter to help me care for the smaller children. She cooks, bathes the younger ones, and helps get them ready for school in the mornings. I don't know what I'd do without her. This decision is so hard, but it's one that I have to make. I have asked God in advance for His forgiveness and because I believe that His word is true, I can proceed with what I need to do."

With chills down my spine I proceeded with the necessary counseling and signing of documents in preparation for her procedure. Because her story was so touching to me, I escorted her into the Operating Room and stayed by her side as she had her procedure done. She chose to have this procedure done under local anesthesia which meant she would be awake with minimal discomfort. She showed no emotion during the time of the procedure, she laid on the table still with her eyes closed. Once done, she broke down crying and again, I held this lady in my arms and we just hugged until she left the operating room. This patient's story touched me in a way that I couldn't imagine, so I gave her my personal phone number and told her to call me whenever she needed to. We stayed in touch for several months, until we lost touch. I don't know how her story ended, but I'm just glad that God put me in that place at that time to be a blessing and a support to her.

CHAPTER 12

Robbed of Her Innocence

"There is no greater evil than those who willingly
hurt innocent children."
Aleesha Poe

It is said that life is the most precious thing given to us by God, and I agree. But I watched a precious little girl undergo general anesthesia surgery to terminate a 15-week pregnancy at the tender age of 9. After she completed the procedure, she was wheeled into the recovery room. She was innocent, small, and sleeping peacefully. I happened to be one of the nurses in the recovery room responsible for her post-operative care. I went outside in the waiting area to give her mom an update of her status and let her know how the surgery went. I did not know this lady at all, only the small amount of information I was given for this surgery. I took her into a private room where we could talk. I assured this mom that I was not here to judge her, but that I was a nurse working in this field and here to serve the very women that cross my path. She thanked me, and we hugged as though we knew each other for years. She appeared so troubled that I could not just walk away so I asked her if she wanted to talk, she said yes and proceeded to tell me her story. Of all the experiences I've had in this field, this story broke my heart the most. This is her story.

This patient's mother received a distraught call from her daughter's guidance counselor at her school while working. Her daughter would not be released until her mother came to retrieve her from school. Once her mother arrived at the school, the guidance counselor handed a note to the child's mother and asked her to read it. The note was retrieved from her daughter while being passed between her and another student during class. The child's teacher had taken the note and when she read it, she escorted the child and her note to the guidance counselor for follow up. The note mentioned that her child was engaging in sexual behavior with her step dad, her mother's husband.

As angry and hurt as the mother was when she read this letter, she was encouraged not to go home but to go to the police department instead, in which, she did. She and her daughter were escorted to the police department where they were counseled separately for a moment. This child's mother was advised that child protective services would have to be contacted and that this report will require immediate investigation. After filing a report with the police department, the mother was recommended to proceed to the hospital so that the child could have a full examination. Once in the emergency room, a social worker, a representative from the Child Protective Services and a forensic nurse greeted mom and her daughter. The child was given a vaginal exam as mom was present to comfort her daughter. Mom later expressed how disturbed she was that her daughter seemed to be "unbothered" by the fact that her daughter was comfortable with the vaginal speculum used for the exam.

After the exam the child was then given a sonogram to rule out a pregnancy or damage to any internal organs. The sonogram revealed a 15-week pregnancy. This infuriated the mother even more. She said she was in complete denial. She could not understand why her husband would do this to her baby girl and to her. Her mother said her daughter never had a period, never showed any signs of pain or discomfort, and never came to her mother to talk about anything. The mother said she never saw any reason to question her daughter because she seemed like a happy 9-year-old girl and her husband treated her daughter like his own child. The mother said she often left her child alone with her husband if she had to run errands but never in a million years expected anything like this to happen. The mother said her daughter's father lived in another state but talked to his daughter often via phone and she never mentioned anything or sounded like she was sad or hurt at any time during their conversations.

After the exam and sonogram were completed the mother and her daughter were interviewed again by the social worker and the Child Protective Services representative along with a female officer. The mother was advised by the representatives to remain quiet so that they could get a full detailed account of what was going on from the child. The mother said she found it so hard to compose herself listening to the graphic details of her daughter's testimony.

The daughter explained that, in the beginning, her stepdad would buy her candy or anything she wanted if she allowed him to touch her and perform oral sex on her. He told her that it would not hurt, but that it would feel good, and that all pretty girls did this. Most times, this took place when mom was not home or when he gave her a bath and prepared her for bed. Eventually the acts elevated, and the daughter was asked to "return the favor" and perform oral sex on her stepdad. When she was comfortable with that, he started rub his genitals against her thighs until eventually he would penetrate her. She told the social worker that initially it hurt but then it didn't hurt anymore. He told her not to tell anyone because if she did 'they' were going to 'kill her mother and her father' so she remained quiet.

The gifts continued, as well as the sex. Eventually the daughter told a friend in school via a note. She wrote in a note, explaining what she and her stepdad did the night before, how it felt, and what reward came from that. This note was then passed to another friend, but never made it to her because the teacher noticed the two girls talking and passing this note. The teacher went over to the girls and asked for the note. Once retrieved, she read it, stopped the class, and escorted the girl to the guidance counselor.

After hearing the testimony of this child, the police went to the victim's house where they apprehended the mother's husband immediately. Several days later the child was brought to the clinic to terminate this pregnancy. Sadly, she was unable to consent because she could not understand what was going to take place. All she knew was that she would go to sleep and wake up with some "tummy pain." This story was the most heartbreaking for me throughout my career.

As the mother of a young daughter at this time, I probably would take the same steps as this mother to terminate this pregnancy. Others may have disagreed but let's just ask the question, If this was your daughter, would you be okay with your 9-year-old innocent daughter carrying a pregnancy by a man who raped her for his own guilty pleasures? Emotionally, mentally, and physically this girl has been scarred enough. For this child to carry a baby that resulted from a traumatic experience is not fair to her. Also, keep in mind the physical danger this child could endure carrying this child. As a pro-life parent, how would deal with this situation?

As heartbreaking as this story was, the specimen was collected for evidence and proved to be an exact match for his DNA. He was sentenced to 10 years in jail for statutory rape, child endangerment, and abuse. Mom eventually divorced him.

CHAPTER 13

Teenagers, My Superheroes

Teenagers are my favorite group of people. They are my "Superheroes" they are invincible, and they "know it all." They are challenging, and they challenge my intellect. I've come across many teenagers in my years as a nurse, and I've always said, "If I can just reach one, I've done my sworn duty as a nurse."

Ms. Thomas, RN

A 16-year-old female came into the clinic, brought by her grandmother. Her behavior toward her grandmother was degrading and rude. I happened to be the nurse counseling this patient at the time. When I was ready to see them, I called them into my room. I asked them each how they are doing, the grandmother responded, but her granddaughter did not. She looked at me, rolled her eyes and sucked her teeth as if I was bothering her. When her grandmother told her to speak, she looked at her grandmother mother and said, "Okay whatever." From this moment, I knew I had a problem child on my hands.

Her grandmother told me she overheard from neighbors that her granddaughter was "raped" into a gang and may be pregnant. She brought her to the clinic to have a pregnancy test and a HIV test. I asked the young lady was this what she was here for and she told me, it wasn't true..."my grandmother is bugging, right now." I asked her if she'd mind being examined and tested, and to my surprise, she agreed. The testing procedure was explained in detail, and then the young lady was asked for a blood and urine sample.

While the patient was in the bathroom, I had a chance to talk with her grandmother. Her grandmother informed me that her granddaughter was the sixth of nine children that her daughter had left behind. Her daughter died from AIDS and she was the only living relative who would take all of her grandchildren in. The grandmother expressed that it was challenging raising all her daughter's children and working full-time to support them. The oldest child was 17 years old and more often than not, she had to rely on her to care for the remainder of the children until she came home from work. The other children were mindful, respectful, and often followed the rules of the house, but this child was rebellious and headed down the wrong road. She skipped school, she was sexually active, and she was very disrespectful. The grandmother said that the neighborhood they lived in did not make matters any better because gangs, drugs and crime populated the area they lived in. The grandmother said that at times she considered placing her granddaughter in foster care. However, she said she could not do that because she knew how corrupt the system was and she did not want that on her conscience. She said she's doing her best, but this child is the most difficult. She said because she loved her grandchildren, she could not give up on them, especially this child. After venting to me, the grandmother, broke down crying in my office. All I could do was hug her and try to convince her that things were going to be okay.

After the young patient returned to the room, I asked her grandmother to step out for a moment and allow me to talk to her granddaughter alone. I was not intimidated by her attitude or "hardcore" look, but I was nervous as to how I was going to get my point across. The only way this would work would be to rid my professionalism and bring myself down to the patient's level. I was extremely firm in my approach and was straight forward.

At first, talking to her was like a talking to a brick wall—nothing penetrated. So, I resorted to a technique I was known for at my job. I showed patients pictures of Sexually Transmitted Infections (STIs) at their worst. This always grossed out my patients, but I'd learned that pictures speak louder than words. So, that's exactly what I did. I pulled out my pictures and soon after, I started to see a shift in her body language and attitude. It worked! I broke through, so I thought. She began to ask questions as if she was concerned and I just kept answering. The more conversation we engaged in, the more I felt obligated to teach her what I knew in preventing her from "looking like" one of those pictures in the book. This session lasted 20 minutes and I felt that maybe, just maybe I was able to break her.

Her pregnancy test confirmed an 8-week pregnancy that day. After giving her test results, I saw a change in her behavior and her eyes began to fill with tears. I asked how she felt and she told me that she did not want a baby. I discussed her options with her and she was scheduled for an abortion 2 days later. I explained the procedure in detail as well as birth control options as she listened closely to what I had to say. After giving her all this information, I asked her if she had any questions and she said, "No I just want to know if you are going to be there in the operating room with me."

I asked, "Why is that?" "Because I am scared," she told me. This tough girl—that was so disrespectful—was now this vulnerable and frightened little girl who needed my help. A part of me felt good because I knew I broke her shell, but a bigger part of me felt bad because she was a vulnerable baby who could be easy persuaded and taken advantage of at any time.

After confirming the pregnancy news with the grandmother, the patient walked out of the office in shame and fear. I assured the grandmother that I would do everything in my power to help her granddaughter through this.

Her STI results would not be back until two weeks later when she would return for follow up. I don't know why, but she stayed on my mind until she came back. She decided to stay awake with local anesthesia and I must say it was a difficult experience for her, one that I'm sure she would remember. I kept my promise and stayed by her side during the entire process.

After the procedure was complete, she broke down crying, not because she was in any physical pain, but because her soul had been broken. When I asked how she felt, she replied, "I never meant for this to happen and I hate that I put my grandmother through so much anguish and grief. I'm going to change my ways and make my grandmother proud of me. I am sorry, I'm sorry, I'm so sorry."

After the procedure, I wrapped my arms around this young lady and asked God to forgive her. I told her, "When we leave this room, it's over and done. If you believe that God has forgiven you, then He has. Let it go." With that she wiped her tears and together we walked out of the operating room. After her recovery, I escorted her to her grandmother and with open arms she hugged her granddaughter and together they cried. The grandmother thanked me for being by her daughter's side, and I whispered in her ear that even superheroes lose their powers sometimes.

In two weeks, this patient returned to the clinic for her postoperative follow up and I was in for the shock of my life. Her grandmother came to my office and asked to speak with me before I saw her granddaughter. She said to me, "Nurse Monica, I don't know what it was you told my grandbaby, but she has made a complete transformation in just 2 short weeks. She's my 'golden child!' What did you say or do?" I told her grandmother that I spoke her granddaughter's language and I showed her the consequences, in pictures, of what could happen if she continues down this path, not to mention being by her side during her abortion. She said, "Well, Nurse Monica, it worked, and I just want to say thank you for everything you've done." Five minutes later this once, *gang-looking, hard-core, attitude-having female* walked into my office. Chills covered my body, because she looked the exact opposite. No attitude, neatly dressed, and very respectable. She hugged me, and I hugged her back and she whispered to me "Thank you."

She was advised by the provider that all was well and she was also free of any STI's. She said she would not be sexually active any more, that school was more important because she wanted to be a nurse just like me, and she wanted to do what I do. I told her that "All things are possible through Christ, who gives us strength." Believe it and it will be done, and I will be there for guidance, if you need me. When she left, I just put my head on my desk and cried, because if I didn't reach any other teenager, I reached ONE. I kept my promise and stayed in touch with this patient. She graduated from high school a year later and started her nursing career at a local NYC college. Three years later she graduated with her Associate's Degree as a Registered Nurse.

"Love yourself enough to set boundaries. Your time and energy are precious. You get to choose how you use it. You teach people how to treat you by deciding what you will and won't accept."

Anna Taylor

CHAPTER 14

Why is God Punishing Me?

"My understanding of God does not permit me to accept that every bad or good thing that occurs is a reward or punishment. There are times when bad things happen to good people."

Jerome Epstein

I provided care to a patient who decided to terminate her pregnancy at 16 weeks. This patient's pregnancy was diagnosed with a fetal abnormality that would cause the fetus to die due to complications after birth. This is her story.

This 46-year old patient was pregnant for the second time after five years. She was a well-educated and studious woman who had decided to secure her career before starting a family. She had been married for 10 years prior to this and once she and her husband were in a financially stable place, they decided to have children. Her first pregnancy had resulted in the birth of her first son. She said she wanted to get pregnant soon after that but when her son was diagnosed with autism at age 2, they decided to wait. She expressed that raising a child with autism was challenging and consumed most of her time and energy. When her son was 5 years old, they decided to get pregnant with their second child. For whatever reason getting pregnant was a challenge for a long while. After a year of trying she finally got pregnant. When she suspected she was pregnant she went to the doctor for confirmation and to her surprised she was further along than she thought, 14 weeks. With this pregnancy she was filled with so much joy and passion that she would have an addition to her family.

84

After her initial prenatal blood work, she was advised of some discrepancies and was told she needed to follow up. She was informed that her pregnancy was diagnosed with a "rare fetal abnormality" and would require additional testing. Not certain what would happen with this pregnancy, she continued to pray and trust in God that everything would be okay. Abortion at this time was not an option for her and her husband. Days seemed like weeks and weeks seemed like years waiting to hear good news. Finally, after two long stressful weeks she was contacted by her obstetrician's office to come in for a sonogram. The sonogram report along with addition testing confirmed a fetal abnormality. Her obstetrician then gave her more devastating news when he told her that not only did her unborn fetus have an abnormality, but it was lethal anomaly that would eventually result in the death of her infant soon after birth. She recalls that she felt as if she was hit with a bag of bricks. Her obstetrician recommended the

85

immediate termination of her pregnancy. She says that her faith in God told her that abortion was not an option and that she should continue her pregnancy as God had ordered. She was perplexed, confused, and faced every emotion that exists. After talking to her husband and praying on it, she decided that in the best interest of their family she would terminate her pregnancy. She came to the clinic seeking an abortion because she could not emotionally carry this child for nine months with all the odds against it. She expressed that this was the hardest decision she had to make but she was ready to move forward with her decision. Nursing doesn't just involve "caring for a patients' needs" it involves having a listening ear, a humble and sincere heart, and most importantly having a character that is not judgmental.

After listening to this patient pour her heart out to me, I felt obligated once again to support her to the very end of this difficult journey. I accompanied her to the OR and was by her side when she awoke. I told her that everything went well, and that God was in control. I leaned in toward her and whispered in her ear a prayer of forgiveness and together we prayed:

Lord we know not why you take us through life's trials and tribulations, but we accept it and get through it. We thank you for life, and we ask that you continue to watch over us. We ask all these things in your name, Amen.

The tears began to flow from both of our eyes and all I could do was to embrace this patient by hugging her. I told her that when you ask God to take control you have to "let go" and do as he says, so when you walk out of the operating room, leave this behind, let go and let God. Now of course I know this is easier said than done but your slate has been wiped clean and you have been forgiven. She said having me by her side made all the difference for her, as she later expressed in a "patient survey report" It made my heart feel good knowing that once again God put me in the right place at the right time.

CHAPTER 15

My Guilty Spirit

"The problem simply put is that we cannot choose everything simultaneously. So, we live in danger of becoming paralyzed by indecision, terrified that every choice might be the wrong choice."

Elizabeth Gilbert

Most women dream of motherhood at some point in their lives. Motherhood is an unbreakable bond between a mother and her child. It is the miracle of life given to us by God for those who believe. It comes with the beautiful experience of knowing that inside of our precious womb is a replica of us.

I know a lady who is very dear to me. She was newly married and immediately decided to start a family. Before her marriage she experienced a pregnancy that resulted in an abortion. She had no medical history and to her knowledge, she was in outstanding health. Who knew that soon after marriage her faith would be tested? For the first 5 years of their marriage, she and her husband tried to conceive unsuccessfully. As her frustration grew, she continuously questioned God.

I can only imagine wanting something as precious as a baby so badly that it kills you inside to know that you can't have one when you want. Needless to say, my dear friend NEVER gave up faith. She believed it would happen when the time was right and not before then. She did not like this, but she accepted it and was patient. Doctor visits became the norm for her and her husband. Her gynecologists told her she had a cyst on her ovaries that may have caused a disturbance in her conception process. After months of counseling, her physician started her on a medication that seemed to be a promising way to help aid her conception.

With the odds against her conceiving naturally, she and her husband decided to give this medication a try. This medication, through studies, proved effective in helping women to conceive by releasing multiple eggs from the ovaries. For several months she faithfully took this medication and prayed for that outcome to be what she had so desired for so long. After five long years of trying, they eventually conceived. It was a dream come true for the young couple, things started to look good and promising, and they were finally happy about having a child.

Knowing that I worked in this field, she confided in me about her new pregnancy and I gave my word to keep it confidential. As weeks went by, life grew inside her body and she began to embrace her pregnancy as most mothers do. I remember our conversation like it was yesterday. I told her I had a dream, and I saw two babies in the dream. We laughed as she told me her recent sonogram revealed only one pregnancy. At this time, she was seven weeks pregnant and the pregnancy was going well. It was only a dream, and whether I was wrong or right, she was carrying a life and I was happy for the young couple. Several weeks into the pregnancy, sadly she suffered a miscarriage. It was a devastating blow but, she had been forewarned by her gynecologists that this could happen. She managed to pull herself together afterwards because giving up was not an option for her. Accepting it for what it was, she remained faithful that one day it would happen when the time was right.

A few weeks later, at approximately 3:00 in the morning, I received a call from my good friend. She was feeling excruciating pain in her lower abdomen and was bleeding. Initially, I was baffled by what could possibly be going on. The miscarriage she just suffered, happened several weeks prior and I did not think this episode related to that episode weeks prior. I knew she told me that only one pregnancy was confirmed but I felt differently about that. I'm not a dream master but my intuition and experience in this field, told me she was pregnant with more than one baby and this baby was not in her uterus but in her fallopian tubes.

I recommended that she go to the hospital immediately for further evaluation. My suspicion was confirmed, she had a ruptured ectopic pregnancy (a pregnancy that develops outside of the uterus, usually in the fallopian tubes). This was the second baby I dreamt about. Not only would she lose the baby, but one of her fallopian tubes as well. This would decrease her chances to conceive by 50%. Saddened by this ordeal, she wanted to give up, but the fighter in her would not let her. She was determined to have her baby, so soon after this ordeal she restarted her prescribed medication and prayed for all the best again. If she was going to give up, she was going to exhaust all her possibilities first. After several months, she found herself pregnant again, but this time she proceeded with caution. After suffering the loss of two pregnancies back to back, she was anxious and unattached. After a few weeks, this pregnancy ultimately resulted in another ectopic pregnancy; this time her body gave signals that "something was wrong" and she decided to investigate sooner, rather than later. Sooner played in her favor, because although this pregnancy also resulted in an ectopic pregnancy, and she was prescribed a medication that would evacuate the pregnancy without damaging her remaining fallopian tube. She realized that the initial medication she was taking to help her conceive, may have been the culprit for these unfortunate pregnancies, so against her doctor's recommendation to continue this medication, she

94

decided to stop taking it. If it was God's will for her to have a child then it would be, and if it wasn't, she would just deal with it. Knowing every bit of this information, my guilt started to kick in. On one hand I had a good friend whose only desire was to be a mother and would go beyond measures to do that. On the other hand, I worked in an environment where abortions were performed daily up to 24 weeks (6 months). At times, I wished I could just breathe life into one of my patients BABIES and just give it to my good friend. After thinking long and hard, I called and had a heart-to-heart conversation with her. I expressed to her my deepest sympathy and offered be a surrogate mother for her and her husband. Due to the nature of my job as a nurse in this field, my conscience haunted me for a long time. After praying on this for a while, my heart and spirit spoke to me and told me to offer this option in exchange for my soul's redemption. Be a blessing to someone that needed a blessing is what I thought. Here I was a single mom

95

with two small children, living check-to-check, willing to sacrifice my body and give life to a woman who desired a child more than anything in the world.

" A kind gesture can reach a wound that only compassion can heal."

Steve Maraboli

She said to me that she was surprised, yet humble and grateful that I would offer to do this for her and her husband. She told me that she was NOT going to give up and that she believed that it would happen one day when the time was right because that's how God works, not when we want it, but when we are ready to receive it.

Approximately four to five months later when we were together, I told her she was pregnant. She looked at me is total surprise and shocked that I knew because, this time the couple did not tell anyone about this new pregnancy. For a split second she thought maybe her husband told me about the pregnancy, but he never did. Once again, this revelation came to me in a dream. In the dream I saw a baby girl wrapped in a red blanket. She was beautiful, healthy and she was due to arrive into this world within days of Valentine's Day. Nine months later my good friend finally got her wish and delivered a healthy baby girl close to Valentine's Day.

"You may feel that God is slow in coming to your rescue or meeting that need you have. But God's timing is perfect, and he is always right on time."

Spiritual Inspirations

CHAPTER 16

Until it's You, You'll Never Understand

Marie was the mother of three beautiful children (ages 10, 7, and 3). Married for nine years, she and her husband were financially in a good place. They were content with the family they had, but believed that children were a blessing, so if they should get pregnant again, they would welcome this child with love and happiness to their family. They were a Christian family and believed that life was the most precious gift from God. Two years after her third child was born Marie was diagnosed with Lupus.

Lupus is an autoimmune disease. With Lupus the immune system attacks the healthy tissues and organs in your body. There is no cure, but people can live a normal lifestyle with daily maintenance. However, Lupus can cause life-threatening complications with the heart, kidneys, and/or other organs of the body in a woman who is pregnant. The women's pregnancy would be deemed high-risk and she would require frequent prenatal monitoring throughout her pregnancy.

With daily maintenance, Marie was able to live a "normal life" since her diagnosis, having only one minor flair up from which she quickly recovered. Several months later, Marie experienced pain in her left leg. With pain medication the discomfort initially subsided, but Marie soon realize that she was taking pain medication several times a day and the pain began to compromise her walking. She visited her rheumatologists who quickly assessed her situation. After testing and exploring

Marie was given the reason for her discomfort. She said the doctor told her she had two issues going on. Marie was given the news that she had a stabilized blood clot in her leg that could be corrected with medication. The second piece of news was that she was pregnant. Marie told me that in a million years she was not ready to hear this news because for the past few years she had been very careful and successful in preventing pregnancy.

After her diagnosis, Marie's rheumatologists advised her to prevent any future pregnancies for the sake of preserving her own health. She was advised to not take hormonal birth control because it would interfere with the medication she was taking to suppress Lupus. Sometimes she and her husband used condoms, but most times, Marie relied on her biological clock—the fertility rhythm method—to keep from getting pregnant. Because she was so successful in this method, she felt confident that she was able to control her body; for five years it worked.

After her last flair up, Marie had her Lupus under control, but her health was fragile and she was still at risk for any life-threatening conditions. As advised by her rheumatologists, pregnancy was one of those life-threatening complications, and she should consider terminating her pregnancy. Although she was surprised about her pregnancy, she was accepting of it and prepared for the challenge. She would do what she needed to have a healthy pregnancy and carry to term. Against the odds, and her doctor's advice, she and her husband decided to continue the pregnancy. Marie did not believe in abortion; she believed that every child's name is written in the *Book of Life* and that God always had the final say. You see, Marie was the wife of a pastor. She was the First Lady of their church and many followed their teachings.

Abortion is what she preached *against* and what she did not promote, so it was not an option.

Sixteen weeks (4 months) into the pregnancy, Marie encountered her first serious complication. She had trouble breathing and was taken to the hospital. After evaluation it was determined that a second blood clot was found in her lung. With her husband by her side they were given the news that her pregnancy was at risk and terminating the pregnancy was recommended to preserve her life. Marie was in a critical life or death situation and a decision had to be made immediately. Against their belief to take an innocent life, they decided to terminate the pregnancy. It was not an easy choice, but it was necessary to save her life.

Marie said terminating her pregnancy was the hardest decision she had to make even with knowing she could lose her life. She said she went through depression for months afterwards. Eventually Marie recovered but she said was happy that she could have the procedure done safely and confidentially. She still believed that abortion was morally wrong, she did not condone abortion but she said since her experience, she has been more understanding and sensitive to women who went through this tragic experience.

CHAPTER 17

A Woman's Rights

A woman's reproductive rights gives her the legal right to make decisions for her reproductive health and the care she receives, including the right to safe and legal abortion, contraception and sexual education, free of judgement.

The choice to abort a pregnancy is NEVER easy, but having a CHOICE is what's even more important. Just imagine if your rights as a woman were taken away and you were forced to carry an undesired pregnancy. How would you feel? What would you do? We cannot ignore the fight and the struggles women before us have made. The Women's Movement prompted a great movement in women's history and we should not let their sacrifices be in vain.

I am a Woman, I am proud, and I am a PRO-CHOICE CHRISTIAN NURSE.